Annihilate Your Acne

How to Get Rid of Acne and Create Beautiful, Clear Skin

Mike Mains

DISCLAIMER

The contents of this book are based upon experience and research conducted by the author. This information is not intended as medical advice, but rather a sharing of knowledge and information from the experience and research of the author. This work is for informational purposes only and is not intended to diagnose or treat any disease. The author and publisher present this information and the reader accepts it with the understanding that anything done or tried as a result from reading this work is at the reader's own risk. The author and publisher shall have neither liability nor responsibility to any person or entity with respect to any loss, damage, or injury caused, or alleged to be caused, directly or indirectly, by the information contained in this work.

Copyright © 2020 by Mike Mains

ISBN: 978-1-953006-09-7 (Paperback)

ISBN: 978-1-953006-06-6 (E-Book)

All Rights Reserved. No part of this book may be reproduced in any manner without the express written consent of the author, except in the case of brief excerpts in critical reviews or articles. The information contained in this book is for educational purposes only. The author and publisher assume no responsibility whatsoever for any loss incurred by any person or business in connection with the information in this book.

Author contact: mainsmike@yahoo.com

Table of Contents

Exciting News For You..1

Chapter One

What No One Else Will Tell You: The True Cause of Acne.....3

Chapter Two

What to Eat and Drink..11

Chapter Three

Sleep Your Acne Away..25

Chapter Four

The Power of Sunlight..29

Chapter Five

The Fluoride Connection..31

Chapter Six

Emotions and Your Health...33

Chapter Seven

Saving Your Soul – Your Ultimate Challenge........................41

Exciting News for You!

I have good news, great news, and fantastic news!

The good news is that before you even finish reading this book you will have a thorough understanding of the true cause of acne. The true cause of acne is something almost no one else will tell you, but I will.

The great news is that in less than one month, based on my experience and provided you make a few simple changes in your life, your acne will already be in retreat and you will be well on your way to glowing and radiant skin.

The fantastic news is that none of this is going to cost you a penny. No snake-oil supplements. No skin-suffocating lotions or creams. No dangerous drugs. No nothing. Just common-sense advice and a few healthy lifestyle choices are all that's needed.

Are you excited? Are you ready to annihilate your acne and begin your path to clear and radiant skin?

With your permission, let's get started.

Note: This is a short and easy-to-read book. Unlike other authors, I have no interest in padding 50 pages of information into 250 pages of useless fluff in order to sell you an over-priced book. I know firsthand the extreme pain you are enduring because of your acne. I was there myself. So rather than bog you down with hundreds of pages and hours of time spent reading, I've distilled the essence of everything you need to know into this quickly-read, easy-to-understand work. In less than an hour of reading, you can be on your way to beautiful and crystal clear skin.

Keeping the page count down also allows me to make this information affordable to virtually everyone, regardless of their financial situation. I can offer the paperback version of this book for less than ten dollars and the E-book version for less than five dollars. What's more, no acne-sufferers will be turned away for lack of funds. If you can't afford five dollars to clear up your acne and create beautiful, clear skin, email me and I will send you the information for free.

Chapter One - What No One Else Will Tell You: The True Cause of Acne

Do you suffer from acne? I did – for many years – until I discovered what causes acne and how to eliminate it. Once I did that, my acne literally melted away. How fast, you ask? In my case, it took two weeks for most of my acne to disappear and about a month before all of it was gone. Your case might be the same or it might be different. But is a month of time really too long to rid your face of unsightly acne and replace it with beautiful, glowing skin?

This book is different from any other book on acne you may have read, and the information it contains is different from the information that any doctor or dermatologist will ever tell you.

The reason this book is different is because I am telling you the truth. Unlike others, I have no financial incentive in perpetuating your acne. I have no drugs, creams, lotions, or products to sell you. (You can read the cleverly disguised comments from those that do sell those things in the review section for this book.)

This book is also different, because it comes with my personal support. You can email me at any time with any questions or concerns you have and I will be happy to answer you. Other authors don't offer personal support, but I do.

I have no axe to grind, no grudge to bear. My only interest is helping you to heal your acne and replace it with beautiful, clear skin. Prepare to blown away by information that no one else is willing to tell you.

Know Your Enemy

The first rule of warfare is Know Your Enemy. The first rule when it comes to annihilating your acne is to know its true cause. Once you know the true cause of acne, then all you need to do is make a few slight pivots in your life to avoid the things that are causing it.

When you stop causing your acne, it literally disappears. That's how it worked for me and that's how it has worked for thousands of others. Sound simple? It is, really.

Let's start with a few common myths and misconceptions.

Misconception #1) Acne is caused by hormones.

At one time, it was fashionable to claim that acne was caused by hormones – it's what I was told when I was a teenager – but I don't think anyone believes this whopper anymore. Science has proven the "acne-is-caused-by-hormones" theory to be false and it has thankfully gone the way of newspapers, pay phones, and VHS movies.

Misconception #2) Acne is caused by glands producing excess oil.

The belief that acne is caused by glands producing excess oil is a common misconception among doctors and dermatologists. They believe it for two reasons. First, because it's what they've been taught. Second, because it provides them with an excuse to sell you unnecessary and expensive drugs, medications, creams and lotions. I feel bad for some of these doctors and dermatologists, because I actually believe they are sincere and truly on a quest to heal acne. They just don't know how to do it.

You can prove to yourself that acne is not caused by glands producing excess oil very easily in two ways. The first way is by looking in the mirror. Is your acne still there? You've been following your doctor and your dermatologist's advice, right? Taking all their medications and slathering your face with their skin-drying lotions and creams, and yet your acne is still there, isn't it? (I know it is or you wouldn't be reading this book.)

What does that tell you? If acne is caused by glands producing excess oil, shouldn't their products that are specifically designed to stop your glands from producing excess oil be working?

The second way to prove that acne is not caused by glands producing too much oil is by taking a quick stroll through history. Do that and you'll quickly discover that acne is a 20th century and 21st century affliction. In other words, before the 20th century, people did not suffer from acne. Did you know that?

Now you'll have to conduct your historical research independently, because there are plenty of liars out there who will tell you otherwise, but prior to the 20th century, there was little to no acne, especially among teenagers.

When David slew Goliath, there was no teenage or adult acne. When Hernan Cortes conquered Mexico, there was no teenage or adult acne. When Shakespeare wrote *Romeo and Juliet*, there was no teenage or adult acne.

Think about that for a moment. If acne was caused by glands producing too much oil (or by hormones), then why wasn't it happening prior to the 20th century?

The answer to that question is a big clue to what really causes acne, which we'll cover in just a few moments.

Misconception #3) Acne is genetic.

Acne is not genetic. If your parents had acne, there's no reason why you should also have acne, unless ... and this is a big unless ... you are following the same lifestyle habits that they are.

Did a bell just go off in your head?

Did you just experience an *Ah-Ha* moment?

Good for you, if you did, because you've just stumbled upon the true cause of acne.

Misconception #4) There is no cure for acne.

The people flouting this misconception almost always have a financial incentive in keeping you clueless. By telling you there is no cure for acne, they are able to sell you their overpriced and dangerous drugs, lotions, and creams as a means of *treatment* for acne, not as a cure.

You see, if their products actually worked, they would cure your acne. Because their products do not work, they tell you there is no cure for acne, only different ways of *treating* it. They use their "no cure" nonsense as an excuse to keep you coming back to them as a repeat customer. It's really quite insidious when you think about it.

The truth is there *is* a cure, not only for acne, but for every disease under the sun. Anyone who tells you otherwise is either a fool or a liar or both. However, the cure for acne does not lie in a pill, cream, or lotion, but in your own body. The human body is self-healing. Provide your body with the necessary elements it needs to repair and rejuvenate and it will heal itself of virtually anything.

Acne is no different. To annihilate your acne all that's required is to stop doing the things that cause acne and start doing the things that your body needs to heal itself of acne. And that is an excellent way for us to introduce the true cause of acne.

The True Cause of Acne

Acne is caused by toxicity in the body.

When the body is overloaded with toxicity it releases that toxicity through the skin in the form of acne.

Because acne is caused from within – toxicity within the body – the way to heal it is also from within. Creams and lotions applied from the outside – the surface of your skin – do not work for that very reason. They attempt to heal an affliction that comes from within through treatment that comes from without.

Drugs do not work either, because they do not remove the toxicity within the body that is causing acne. In fact, drugs make things worse by increasing toxicity in the body.

When someone tells you that acne – or any illness – is incurable, they are lying to you. However, hidden within their words is a truth they don't realize is there. Separate the first syllable of the word "incurable" from the rest of the word and here's what you get: in-curable.

Take a look at that word: "in-curable." It tells you that illness is curable, only you have to go with*in* to do it.

The Amazing Power of Your Skin

Did you know that your skin is your body's largest eliminative organ? It's true.

The body is self-healing and always working to keep you in a state of optimum health. Your body can tolerate a little toxicity, but if it becomes overloaded, it will do everything it can to release and cleanse itself of that toxicity.

If your body is unable to release toxicity through the usual channels – sweat, urine, feces, mucus (a runny nose), etc. – it will release that toxicity through the skin. In some people, this takes the form of a rash. In others, hives. And in still others, acne.

Now does it make sense to you?

Acne, along with every other disease, is caused by toxicity in the body. It is a lifestyle affliction. By that I mean it is caused by how we eat, drink, think, behave and worship God. Those are the factors that create toxicity in the body.

It's not your hormones that are causing your acne. It's not your glands secreting too much oil that is causing your acne. And it's not your parents' acne that is causing your acne. It's your lifestyle choices. Those lifestyle choices create toxicity in the body, and your body's efforts to release that toxicity is what causes your acne.

The lifestyle choices that most contribute to your acne are the foods you eat and the beverages you drink. Environmental factors also play a part, as well as your sleeping patterns, your emotions, how you think, and your relationship with God. We'll cover all of those factors in this book.

Now here's the best part about all of this. Since acne is a lifestyle affliction, it means it is totally under your control. You can annihilate your acne and replace it with beautiful, clear skin by making a few simple lifestyle changes.

Change what you're eating and drinking, change your environmental situation, change how you react emotionally, change how you think, change your relationship with God, and almost instantly the appearance of your skin will also change.

Isn't that exciting news? It means the condition of your skin is entirely in your hands. You can change the way your skin looks, and you can do it very rapidly. It won't happen on its own. There are some steps you have to take, but the steps are very easy and we'll walk our way through them together in the pages of this book. The pace is entirely up to you.

You can take baby steps, making only small, incremental lifestyle changes, or you can jump in feet-first. If you choose the former – baby steps - it will take longer for your body and your skin to heal, but you will get there eventually.

Look at it this way: You can travel from Los Angeles to San Francisco by car, or you can travel by foot. One method of travel is faster than the other, but in either case, you'll eventually arrive in San Francisco, even if you only take one step a day.

It's the same when your goal is reducing toxicity in the body and healing acne. You can proceed slowly or you can proceed quickly, but the end result will be the same: your body will heal, your acne will shrivel away, and your skin will look radiant and beautiful.

The speed at which you progress is entirely up to you.

Are you ready to get started? Just say the word, because if you're ready to start, so am I.

Chapter Two - What to Eat and Drink

When it comes to getting rid of acne, it's less about what you do eat and drink than what you don't eat and drink. To reduce toxicity in your body, it's necessary to eliminate all processed food and beverages. Processed food and beverages contain chemicals, pesticides, and preservatives. These are all foreign to your body. The moment you ingest a foreign substance, your body begins to immediately expel it, in whatever way it can. And one of those ways is through your skin.

The first step in annihilating your acne is to not eat or drink anything that comes in a bag, box, can, jar, bottle, or wrapper. Don't eat fast food, junk food, or restaurant food. Don't eat non-organic fruits or vegetables that have been sprayed with pesticides. Don't consume pasteurized dairy products. Don't eat farm-raised fish or meat that doesn't come from grass-fed animals.

What else is on the verboten list?

No bread. No rice. No grains.

No sandwiches or sandwich meat.

No hamburgers. No French fries. No hot dogs.

No pizza. No cereal. No white flour of any sort.

No coffee. No tea. No soda or soft drinks.

No cookies. No cake. No ice cream.

No snack foods. No gum. No candy.

No seedless fruit except bananas. No jelly. No mustard or ketchup.

No tap water – not for drinking, not for cooking, not for brushing your teeth, not for washing your face. Use distilled water.

No aluminum cookware, only stainless steel.

No microwaved food. Throw your microwave in the trash.

No drugs, lotions or creams.

No sunscreen. No sunglasses. No makeup.

No toothpaste that contains fluoride. (We'll talk more about fluoride in a future chapter.)

No sugar. This is essential if you want to eliminate acne.

That's a pretty extensive list of things not to eat or drink. And right now you're probably thinking of quitting this journey before you even start. Don't do it. Don't quit without at least trying to clear your skin. If you give up now, you are a quitter. Quitters never win, and winners never quit.

What's more, I believe you can do it. I have faith in you, and I'm here to walk with you every step of the way. You can email me for support at any time. You can ask me any question you have. I'm here to help you.

The human body was not designed to consume any of the items listed above. Remember what we said earlier about your body needing to eliminate toxicity? When you consume the foods and beverages listed above you force your body to expel the chemicals, pesticides, and preservatives they contain.

Here's an analogy for you. Suppose you were standing in the center of a hole that you were digging. The first step in getting out of that hole is to put the shovel down and stop digging. Similarly, the first step in eliminating toxicity and allowing your skin to heal and clear is to stop putting toxicity into your body. Makes sense, doesn't it?

Eliminating all of the products listed above is a big first step in clearing up your acne. A *huge* first step. What's more, it's not hard or unpleasant. The truth is once you begin eliminating unhealthy foods and drinks from your life and replacing them with healthy foods and drinks you will love the taste. You will love it so much you will never go back to processed food again. I absolute guarantee it.

You haven't lived until you've eaten a slice of cold, seeded watermelon, or taken a bite from a perfectly ripe banana with little brown spots on the peel, or eaten a chilled cherimoya, the ice cream fruit. (Yes, it is a fruit and, yes, it does taste exactly like ice cream.)

Wild salmon eaten raw or grilled and served with vegetables and/or a salad is absolutely delicious. Beef from grass-fed animals tastes amazing. Raw milk with some raw cream mixed in tastes so good it's almost impossible to stop drinking. (Unfortunately, it's also very hard to find unless you live in California.)

Here's what you can eat and drink: wild, ocean-caught salmon and tuna (not canned), meat from grass-fed animals, organically grown fruits and vegetables (make sure your fruit contains seeds), raw milk and dairy products (available in only a handful of states, so you're probably out of luck), distilled water with organic lemon juice squeezed in, homemade vegetable and fruit juices made with organic produce. Bananas and avocados are possible exceptions to the organic rule as they both have thick protective skins.

That's a short list compared with the do-not-have list, but within it is infinite variety. And within that list are nutritionally rich foods that will strengthen and beautify your body and your skin. Instead of overloading your body with toxicity, you will be flooding it with rich, blood-building nutrition.

If you're wondering where to get wild, ocean-caught fish, grass-fed meat, organic produce, and all the rest, try your local grocery store first. They might surprise you. Farmer's markets are another choice and most communities have them. Health food stores are another option.

When you buy produce, look at the little numbered sticker. If you see a five-digit number, beginning with the number 9, then that produce is organic. That's what you want.

If you see a four-digit number, beginning with the number 4, then that produce is conventional, which means it was grown with pesticides. That's what you don't want.

If you see a five-digit number, beginning with the number 8, then that produce is Genetically Modified. That's what you absolutely do not want, under any circumstances. Almost all potatoes today are GMO. So never eat restaurant potatoes, and never buy and eat potatoes unless you know for a fact that they are organic.

Now if you're really strapped, if you live out in the boondocks and literally have no sources for organic produce, then – and only then – you will have to make do with what you have. In other words, you will have to settle for produce that is not organic. But make sure you soak and wash it to remove as much pesticide as possible. One way to do that is to add a quarter cup of 3% food-grade hydrogen peroxide to a gallon of cold water and soak your produce in it. For leafy vegetables, 15-20 minutes should be enough. For thick-skinned fruits and vegetables, soak them for 30-35 minutes.

Soaking non-organic produce is not the preferable approach, but if that's your only option, go ahead and do it. Just make sure you avoid the other items on the do-not-eat-or-drink list.

Conventional produce with peels, like bananas and oranges, are not as bad as produce without peels, like apples and grapes. I eat conventional Dole bananas on occasion, as well as conventional avocadoes and conventional broccoli that has been well rinsed or soaked. But they're never my first choice. If you're on a quest to annihilate acne, you may want to avoid them.

All of this is going to take a little effort on your part. It's not always easy to find healthy food sources, but it can be done. If your parents aren't willing to help, you'll simply have to do it on your own. After all, it's your skin, not theirs.

My experience is most parents don't want to see their children suffering from acne and would like to help them get rid of it, but they don't know how. Because they don't know how to help, they either do nothing or they commit to a regimen of drugs, lotions, and creams, which only makes things worse.

Other parents are too busy to help. They will tell you they do not have the time to shop for the kind of food you need in order to make your acne disappear. If your parents are like that it doesn't mean they don't love you. Of course, they love you. But they have their own lives to lead, their own pursuits to follow.

You can try explaining to them how the body is self-healing and why you need organic produce, ocean-caught fish, meat from grass-fed animals, and fluoride-free water in order to heal your skin. But don't be surprised if it falls on deaf ears. Most people, including parents, are simply unwilling to listen to logic. Trying to explain logic to people who are unwilling to listen to logic is an endeavor you're going to experience your entire adult life, so you might as well get used to it.

The bottom line regarding parents is if they are willing to help you, fantastic. If not, that's fantastic too. You can look on the situation as a marvelous opportunity to become self-sufficient. That alone will put you ahead of the majority of adults in the world, and far ahead of almost all of your peers. It means you will be responsible for choosing, buying, and preparing almost all of your own meals. If that's the case, so be it. I did it (at age 14), so can you.

The reason for using distilled water is the same as avoiding processed food. Tap water and almost every brand of bottled water contain fluoride and other chemicals. You don't want fluoride or other chemicals anywhere in or on your body. So use distilled water only to brush your teeth and wash your face. Put some into a little spray bottle and spray it on your face or on your toothbrush. For guys, use distilled water for shaving, and avoid shaving cream. Use either distilled water only or use natural soap with no chemicals to shave your face.

You can squeeze some organic lemon juice into distilled water for drinking. And always use distilled water for cooking, never use tap water. Almost every drugstore and grocery store in the country sells distilled water.

Practice Proper Food Combining

Practice proper food combining when eating. Protein, starches, and fruit require different enzymes in order to digest properly. For that reason, consume fruits or fruit juice alone, at least one hour before consuming any other type of food. Two hours before is better. Consume starches alone, although if you have acne, you should avoid all starches, except organic potatoes. You can eat protein, such as meat or fish, with vegetables, but not with fruits or starches. The lone exception might be organic potatoes mixed in with beef stew. Consume vegetable juices alone. Consume raw dairy products alone.

If you ignore proper food combining, your body will have great difficulty digesting your meals. If that happens, you've just created toxicity in your body, and you know what the next step is, right? Your body will begin releasing that toxicity in whatever way it can, most likely through your skin.

Do not drink with your meals. Drinking liquid when you eat causes bloating and makes it hard for your body to digest food. Instead, drink between meals. Drink distilled water with organic lemon juice squeezed in at least three hours after a meal (four hours is better), and at least 30 minutes before a meal (1 hour is better). And drink a lot of water. It will help your body flush out toxicity.

Eat your food slowly and sip your liquids slowly. This is important. Slow eating means a lot of chewing, as well as putting your fork down between bites. This will make it a lot easier for your body to digest what you are consuming. If you shovel food into your mouth, take a couple of token bites, and then swallow it down, your digestion will be severely impaired. Sadly, that's the way most people eat.

Sip your liquids slowly for the same reason.

Whether eating or drinking, relax and think pleasant thoughts. If you're tense, excited, or otherwise emotionally worked up, it's hard for your body to digest food.

What about supplements, you ask? There are only two that I recommend at this point: Vitamin C powder made from organic food sources, such as acerola cherry, NOT ascorbic acid; and fermented cod liver oil with X Factor Gold Concentrated Butter Oil.

If you can't afford those two items, don't worry about it. They're helpful, but not necessary. I didn't have them when I healed my acne. I might have healed my acne faster if I did have them, but that's speculation. If you want to try those supplements, but can't find them, email me and I'll clue you in.

If all of this nutritional talk interests you and you want to delve into the subject further, there's a marvelous book called *Nutrition and Physical Degeneration* by Dr. Weston Price. It might be available at your local library.

Dr. Price was a dentist who traveled around the world in the 1930s, studying the teeth and general health of indigenous people (people native to a land). What he found was startling: indigenous people, eating a natural diet with no processed food whatsoever, had excellent dental health and strong, physically fit bodies.

They had no cancer, no heart disease, no arthritis, none of the diseases that plague modern society. They also had no acne. Many of their communities had no police department or jail, because there was no need for them. Nobody committed any crimes. However, when they began eating processed food, brought in by explorers and settlers, everything changed.

Their health deteriorated rapidly. Crime and delinquency suddenly became problems. Cancer, heart disease, acne, and other illnesses that had been non-existent before, instantly appeared. The same food that most Americans consume on a daily basis destroyed these people. Don't let that happen to you.

If you want beautiful, clear skin, perfect teeth, and a strong and healthy body, then one of the best pieces of advice I can give you is to read Dr. Price's book and follow his diet recommendations. There's only one problem. The book is extremely long and makes for pretty stiff reading.

A far more efficient way to absorb Dr. Price's research is to go online, do a search for his name, and visit the various websites dedicated to him, such as www.price-pottenger.org and www.westonaprice.org.

The absolute best way to learn about Dr. Price and his work is to read the book *Cure Tooth Decay* by Ramiel Nagel, available on the internet. It's an excellent summary of Dr. Price's work and it is extremely easy to read. Everything that book says about eating to improve your teeth also applies to acne and your skin. In fact, it applies to every illness.

If your parents are giving you a hard time about the kind of food you want to eat, give them a copy of *Cure Tooth Decay*, so they can study the research themselves. As I write this, the book is currently selling for around $20. You can probably get a used copy for less than that.

You now know the basics of healthy eating for your skin. If you really want to accelerate your progress, try juicing.

Juicing Will Beautify Your Skin

One thing anyone who wants to improve their health can start doing immediately is juicing. When I talk about juicing, I'm referring to juice you make at home with your own juicer, not any kind of bottled juice available in a store.

Juicing will give you healthier, more vibrant-looking hair, radiant skin, and stronger nails. Who wouldn't want any of those things?

Juicing will also help clear up your acne. It will do that in two ways. First, by helping to detoxify your body. And second, by flooding your body with first-class, easily-absorbable, nutrient-dense nutrition.

Consuming large quantities of fresh, raw, organic vegetable juice is the fastest, easiest, and most effective way to transform both your appearance and your health.

When you juice, you take in large quantities of vitamins, minerals, and live enzymes. It's the quickest way possible to super-charge your body with massive nourishment.

Now imagine what all of those life-affirming nutrients are going to do for your appearance. I'll tell you exactly what they're going to do: your skin will glow, your hair will shine, and your nails will grow clear and beautiful.

I have seen men and women of all ages with haggard-looking skin, weary from life and all of its challenges, begin a serious juicing routine and become so beautiful they were almost unrecognizable.

I've seen dull eyes regain their sparkle, gray hair restored to its original color, and pasty skin rebound with a healthy glow. I've seen people who juice, and others of the same age who opt for plastic surgery, and the juicers look ten to twenty years younger than the face-lifters at a fraction of the cost.

Have you ever noticed the beauty and vibrancy of fruits and vegetables; their bright colors, intoxicating scents, and pulsing life? When you juice, you partake of all the healing qualities and all the phytonutrients that God bestowed upon nature. How can that not reflect itself back in the beauty of your own skin?

Fresh juice is a natural blood-builder. There is nothing, absolutely nothing, you can do to improve both your appearance and your health faster and more efficiently than juicing.

When you juice, you separate the mineral elements from the fiber, leaving only liquid nourishment that your body digests almost instantly. If I was ill, or still had acne, the first thing I would do is begin drinking large quantities of raw, organic vegetable juice.

When that first sip of mineral-rich juice touches your lips, you'll feel a jolt in every cell of your body. The nutrient-dense, life-creating enzymes in the juice will saturate your body and light up your cells with vitality and life. When you juice, you're building beauty and creating clear skin from the inside out.

Norman Walker says, "Vegetable juices are the builders and regenerators of the body. They contain all the amino acids, minerals, salts, enzymes, and vitamins needed by the human body, provided they are used fresh, raw, and without preservatives."

Feeling depressed? Juicing will snap you right out of it. It is impossible to feel any kind of negative emotion when you flood your body with oxygen and nutrients from delicious organic vegetable juice.

Want more energy? Juicing will give it to you. Once you start, you'll wonder how you ever got along without it. In his book *There Are No Incurable Diseases*, the author Dr. Richard Schulze writes about being on the 28th day of a 30-day juice fast: "I was supposed to drive an hour to a gym and kick-box, which takes a lot of energy, much more than regular boxing. I didn't feel up to it. I felt out of energy, but I dragged myself there anyway. After pushing myself through 30 minutes of warm-up exercises it was like I was suddenly on rocket fuel instead of juice. I kick-boxed 17 three-minute rounds. I was better than ever, a personal best. When it was all over, one of the top instructors came over to me and said, "I don't know what you're on, but you were moving so fast we could hardly see you! You were moving so fast you were like a blur!"

(Note: Don't attempt a 30-day juice fast unless and until you are very experienced with juicing!)

Juice carrots, celery, cucumbers, lettuce and bell peppers of all colors. Juice cruciferous vegetables like broccoli and cauliflower. Juice carrots and dandelion together. Juice apples with a slice of lemon and a pinch of ginger. One of the great joys of juicing is discovering different combinations to juice. So experiment and find your own personal favorites. My favorites are celery and cucumber, each juiced separately. It won't be long before you have your own favorites.

If you want beautiful smooth skin, free from acne and blemishes, start juicing today. I guarantee you people will begin to notice and compliment your new and improved appearance. If you're single, you may not be single for long. If you're married, your spouse will fall in love with you all over again. I don't care how bad your acne is or how unattractive you think you might be, start juicing and you'll create a beauty greater than any person you can name.

Juicing doesn't have to be expensive. It can be, but it doesn't have to be. The Rolls Royce of juicers is the Norwalk Juicer, named after Norman Walker, whom we quoted above. That juicer is expensive, but it's also the best. If you are a multi-millionaire, that's the one I would recommend. For the rest of us, you can get along just fine with a Hamilton Beach juicer for around fifty bucks. That's the one I'm currently using, model #67608Z. It's super easy to use and clean. When I started out, I used a Juiceman Jr. juicer, which cost around $40.

Are there any drawbacks to juicing, any at all? Only one I can think of: juicing will increase your need to urinate. For that reason, I wouldn't advise doing it before school or before any other type of social event. However, there's no reason why you can't do it when you are home for the night and/or on the weekends.

It's best to juice on an empty stomach. First thing in the morning is a great time, and also between meals.

Liver – Nature's Super Food

Beef liver from grass-fed animals is nature's super food. It is nature's multi-vitamin, the most nutritious food on the planet. Raw liver (frozen for at least two weeks) from clean sources can restore energy and vitality to even the most exhausted organism.

Liver has an anti-fatigue factor that no other food possesses. It contains more nutrients, gram for gram, than any other food. Dr. Nicholas Gonzalez, a doctor who helps heal cancer holistically, prescribes raw liver to all of his patients. If liver is so good for your health and your body, imagine what it will do for your skin?

You might not like the taste of liver – I didn't, at first – but once you get used to it, it is absolutely delicious. I buy frozen grass-fed liver at Whole Foods.

We're about halfway through this book, but you already have almost everything you need to annihilate your acne and create beautiful skin. The bottom line is to eat *real* food in a calm and tranquil setting, and avoid any and all processed food. With these steps alone, you can heal your acne and replace it with clear, radiant skin.

When I healed my acne – and my acne was *bad* – I had less information than you have now. But I cleared it up completely by changing what I was eating and drinking. Mainly be eliminating all processed and packaged food and replacing it with real food.

What follows next are additional steps you can take to accelerate your progress. I believe they will help you tremendously. They will also enrich your life. Consider them my gift to you.

Chapter Three - Sleep Your Acne Away

Is it really possible to sleep your acne away? You bet it is.

Tissue growth occurs when you sleep and only when you sleep. It actually occurs during the REM (Rapid Eye Movement) phase of sleeping. REM sleep is when you are dreaming and the more you sleep, the more REM phase you experience. During the REM phase of sleeping, your body repairs, recharges, revitalizes, and grows.

That's where the expression "beauty sleep" comes from. The more a person sleeps, the more their skin revitalizes and beautifies. Simply put, the more you sleep, the better you look.

HGH (Human Growth Hormone) is released primarily when you sleep. HGH promotes tissue repair and skin rejuvenation. If you want HGH to do its part in clearing up your skin, be sure to get plenty of sleep.

For athletes reading this, be aware that muscle growth occurs when you sleep. Your muscles don't grow when you are awake and they don't grow when you are exercising; they grow when you are sleeping. If you're working out, you want to be sure and get lots of sleep.

For guys, sleep is a natural alternative to steroids. In fact, old-time bodybuilding coaches used to recommend sleeping after a workout. They called it a "muscle nap" and the prescription was workout, consume nutritious protein, and take a nap. That's not always practical in the real world, but if you can do it, why not? The truth is the more you sleep, the faster your muscles will grow and the quicker your entire body will heal, including your acne.

Personally, I function best with ten hours of sleep a night. You might need a little more or a little less. If you have acne and you're trying to clear it up, I would recommend eight to nine hours of sleep a night as the bare minimum.

When you sleep is almost as important as the quantity of sleep you get. There are certain growth processes that occur in the body from 10 PM till 2 AM that don't occur at any other time, and they only take place when you are sleeping, not when you are awake. So you have to be asleep during those hours in order to benefit.

There are other processes that occur from 2 AM to 6 AM. Again, you have to be asleep during those hours for those growth processes to occur. They won't happen if you are awake.

In order to give your body all of the ammunition it needs to eliminate acne and produce beautiful, clear skin, it's important for you to be in bed and sleeping every night from 10 PM to 6 AM. Even better would be to sleep from 9 PM to 7 AM.

Sleep is one of the most important things you can do for your body. Rest is also important, but not as much as old-fashioned sleep.

Did you know that sleep deprivation is a form of torture? It's true. If you want to drive a person crazy, the easiest way to do that is to deprive that person of sleep.

Unfortunately, almost the entire adult population of the world is chronically sleep-deprived. Not to the extreme that would be labeled torture, but certainly enough to create disease in the body, and certainly enough to prevent the body from operating at peak efficiency.

Sleep helps with depression. There's no better way than sleep to escape from your troubles, for a limited time, anyway.

If you have trouble falling asleep, here's a great tip: try eliminating all sound, starting thirty minutes before you go to bed. By that, I mean no talking, no listening to someone else talk, no music, no television, no sound at all. Your mind will quiet down considerably and you'll find it easy to nod off and enjoy a restful night's sleep.

Also, make sure your bed is comfortable and your room is quiet. If your neighbors are noisy and refuse to quiet down, you have two choices: you can move or you can buy a $20 box fan. Place the fan near your bed and aim it at the wall so it's not blowing all over you. Your purpose in buying the fan is to create ambient noise. The quiet whir of the fan will do that. Hopefully, it will be enough to drown out your neighbors. The fan for this purpose is the 20 inch box fan made by Lasko.

If you have trouble keeping light out of your bedroom, invest in an inexpensive sleep mask. It will deepen your sleep by blocking out all light. Your skin will thank you. Remember, your skin grows, repairs, and regenerates while you are sleeping.

Modern life is difficult, so it might not be possible for you to always get the proper amount of sleep. If that's the case with you, do the best you can. It's the same with your nutritional program: do the best you can with what you have.

No one ever gets it perfect all the time, so take comfort knowing that a little improvement is better than no improvement. And remember our earlier analogy about walking from Los

Angeles to San Francisco? Eventually, you'll get there, even if you only take one step a day.

Eventually, your acne will clear up as long as you continue taking steps in the right direction.

Chapter Four - The Power of Sunlight

Sunlight? Yes, you need it. It's one of the greatest tools at your disposal for creating beautiful, radiant skin. The key, though, is not to wear makeup, sunscreen or sunglasses. Let the healing rays of the sun lovingly touch your skin. Start with five minutes a day and gradually increase up to fifteen or twenty minutes a day.

The best times to sunbathe are early in the morning, from 6-8 AM, or early in the evening, from 5-7 PM. At those times, you get the cooling rays of the sun.

Without sunlight all life on the planet would die. Think about that for a moment and then ask yourself if you really want to spend all your time locked up indoors?

Sunlight boosts your immune system and will help clear up your acne, especially if you have acne on your shoulders or back.

Sunlight decreases stress and is great for healing depression. It's almost impossible to feel depressed when you're under the warm, healing rays of the sun. Have you ever wondered why people get depressed when it rains? It's because they can't see the sun or feel its warm rays on their skin.

Sunlight is excellent for your vision too. If you wear glasses or contacts, spend some time walking around outside without them. You'll notice something amazing happening. Your vision will begin to clear up.

You'll also notice that you can see much better outside in the sun than inside.

Have you ever heard the expression "eagle eye"? It means a person with excellent vision, and it comes from the fact that eagles have excellent eyesight. The reason eagles have excellent eyesight is because they fly high in the sky, with their eyes exposed to the sun, and when they swoop down to pluck a fish from the sea their eyes are exposed to sunlight reflecting off the water.

For more tips on improving your vision, feel free to contact me. (And you thought this book was only about skin care.)

Sunlight is a great source of Vitamin D, an essential nutrient.

If you can sunbathe your entire body, go for it. If not, don't worry about it. Just go for a stroll in the early morning or the very late afternoon and let the sun kiss your skin. Your acne will clear up very fast.

Chapter Five – The Fluoride Connection

How important is the subject of fluoride when it comes to annihilating acne? Very important. Some authors have written entire books about it. Melissa Gallico's book *The Hidden Cause of Acne* is the best. In fact, it's one of the best books ever written about acne, period. If you want a deeper understanding of what causes acne, I recommend reading it. If you're too lazy to read it or you simply don't have the time, I'll sum up its contents right here: fluoride causes acne.

I stumbled upon the fluoride connection to acne when I was a teenager. I couldn't articulate it well, but I knew that tap water, which was heavily fluoridated where I lived, was contributing to my acne. I also noticed that friends of mine who had fluoride treatments performed on their teeth by dentists had horrible acne-ridden skin. Their skin was fine before the fluoride treatments, but broke out immediately afterwards.

A couple of years later, I discovered that fluoride was a waste product of the aluminum industry and actually a poison. Remember what we said at the very beginning of this book about the body needing to release and cleanse itself of toxicity? Well, fluoride is a foreign substance - a poison, no less.

When you consume fluoride in any form, whether by drinking fluoridated water, cooking with fluoridated water, using fluoride toothpaste, putting anything on your skin that contains fluoride, etc., your body immediately begins to release it.

If your body can't release toxicity through the regular channels, it will release it through your skin, your body's largest eliminative organ. In that sense, fluoride is a major cause of acne.

This is why it's so important to use only distilled water and why you need to completely remove fluoride from your life in order to annihilate your acne. Ideally, that includes not showering or bathing in fluoridated water. The trouble there, however, is that very few shower filters remove fluoride. In fact, I've never been able to find one. So this falls into the "do the best you can" area. Take short showers, not long ones, and use distilled water when you wash your face. For guys, use distilled water when you shave your face.

As long as you're dealing with acne, I would also recommend avoiding hot tubs and swimming pools. The water they contain is almost guaranteed to contain fluoride. Do you really want to submerge your body in fluoridated water?

Here's an easy way to avoid using fluoridated water on your face: keep a small spray bottle of distilled water in the bathroom. (You can buy spray bottles for a dollar or less at almost any drug store.) When you brush your teeth, spray some of that distilled water on your toothbrush. (Note: Do NOT use any toothpaste that contains fluoride.) Use that same spray bottle when you wash your face and when you shave. That's all there is to it.

Chapter Six - Emotions and Your Health

Are you surprised to learn there's a correlation between your emotions and your health, or in this case, between your emotions and the condition of your skin? You shouldn't be. It's something that people have always known. It's only in the last one hundred years or so that we've forgotten.

Have you ever heard the expressions "green with envy" or "seeing red"? Those expressions are hundreds of years old. The emotion of envy corresponds to the gallbladder, which is green in color. The emotion of anger corresponds to the liver, which is red in color. When a person experiences envy, they debilitate their gallbladder. When a person experiences anger, they debilitate their liver. Anger can cause a person's skin to erupt in rashes or acne. It can also affect a person's vision.

Have you ever heard someone say, "I was so angry I couldn't see straight"? That's because anger corresponds to the liver, which affects the vision. Almost all vision problems originate in childhood trauma. The child sees or experiences something that is so disturbing he literally distorts his vision in order to block it out of his sight.

That doesn't mean the child was abused, necessarily. He may have lost a pet, or watched something violent on television, or had an embarrassing experience at school.

If you wear glasses or contact lenses, think back to when you first began wearing them. Did you experience some sort of emotional upheaval at the time? Was there something going on in your life – arguing or fighting between your parents, perhaps – that you didn't want to see? I would bet money that the answer is yes.

Old time physicians were much more attuned to the relationship between emotions and health than today's drug pushers. In the old days people with debilitating illnesses were sent to sanitariums out in the country. In those tranquil settings, far from the hustle and bustle of city life and its daily problems, their bodies had a chance to rest and recuperate.

If we still did that today, many people would heal themselves of many different illnesses. Instead, they're drugged up and sent home to die.

Stress can turn hair gray and cause premature aging. If you have ever looked at the photographs of presidents before and after their time in office, the difference is startling. The enormous pressure and responsibility of running the country takes an enormous toll on their appearance. Throw in the fact that almost all of them were corrupt and evil men and it's no wonder that so many of them appeared to age twenty years or more during only four to eight years in office. The lone exception appears to be Ronald Reagan.

Pushed to the extreme, negative emotions can be fatal. Sudden shock or fright can cause a heart attack and actually kill a person.

Just as negative emotions have a debilitating effect on the body and create toxicity, positive emotions have an uplifting effect on the body and contribute to good health. One famous case involves the writer Norman Cousins. He was diagnosed with cancer and cured himself with laughter. Yes, you read that right. He literally laughed his way to health by using humor to cure his cancer.

Cousins knew that negative emotions were contributing to his cancer, so he began watching old comedy movies. Hours of them. He spent his days laughing, which stimulated his immune system, and very soon his cancer was gone. It was so extraordinary he wrote a book about it called *Anatomy of An Illness*.

Louise Hay is another author who healed her illness using positive emotions. Like Cousins, she was diagnosed with cancer and set out to heal herself. Louise didn't use laughter like Cousins did, but she did use positive emotions, positive affirmations, and positive thinking as the basis for her therapy. Like Cousins, she succeeded in completely healing her cancer. Like Cousins, she also wrote a book about it called *You Can Heal Your Life*. (Note: I do not recommend reading either book from these two authors, because in addition to the healing advice they contain, they also allude to or contain false spiritual advice, and Louise's book contains a lot of sinful, negative advice. I mention the titles here for reference only.)

Emotions not only affect our health, they also affect our appearance. Bitter, angry, and resentful people often age more rapidly than others. Their stored up anger and guilt overwhelms the function of their liver and other organs and their skin takes on a sick and sallow complexion.

On the other hand, those who practice forgiveness and cultivate positive emotions often retain a youthful appearance well into middle age and often into their 70s and 80s. Amazing, isn't it?

For our purposes, we want to control our emotional state in order to help heal acne. A good place to start is with humor.

Humor is very healing; just ask Norman Cousins. Did you know that it's impossible to feel anger towards a person with whom you've just shared a laugh? It's true. If there's someone in your life you can't stand, try telling them a joke or some kind of humorous remark the next time you see them. That suppressed smile; that little bit of laughter your words manage to evoke from that person will go a long way toward healing your relationship with them.

I recommend you get your hands on a good joke book (a *good* joke book, I said, not a stupid one), pick out a dozen or so of the funniest jokes, and memorize them. Then start using them. You can also find jokes for free on the internet and you can make up your own. I make up a lot of my own jokes. (Shameless plug: I have a book called *Monkey Jokes: A Joke Book for Kids!* you might find useful, and I have plans to do second book of jokes.)

Keep your jokes clean and funny. The laughter you bring out in others and the laughter you experience for yourself will go a long way toward healing your body. Unfortunately, I cannot recommend any funny movies or comedians, because almost none of them are actually funny. Instead, create your own humor.

In addition to humor, you will find it good for your skin to engage in positive thoughts. If someone has wronged you in the past (or in the present), forgive that person. That doesn't mean to forgo justice. If a person has committed a crime against you, it's important that you continue to seek justice and perhaps jail time for that person. But don't hold a grudge. Don't hold resentment toward them.

Forgive everyone from your past, including and especially the person you find it most difficult to forgive. Ha! That one hurts, doesn't it? Unfortunately (or not), your forgiveness of that person is necessary for your own emotional healing. When you refuse to forgive someone, you're basically allowing that person to continue to harm you. Think about that. Why would you want to continue to experience pain from someone in your past? Forgive and let go. But don't forget, lest you get hurt again.

Practicing forgiveness and focusing on positive thoughts does not mean you will never experience anger. In fact, anger is a necessary emotion. You want to feel anger when you witness injustice and especially when confronted with evil. Psalm 97 says, "Ye that love the LORD hate evil." That's one of the most important sentences in the entire Bible. When you witness evil, you want to feel anger; righteous anger.

Saint Thomas Aquinas, one of the wisest men in the history of the world, said, "He who is not angry when there is just cause for anger is immoral. Why? Because anger looks to the good of justice. And if you can live amid injustice without anger, you are immoral as well as unjust."

Saint John Chrysostom, another great wise man, said, "He who is not angry, whereas he has cause to be, sins. For unreasonable patience is the hotbed of many vices, it fosters negligence, and incites not only the wicked but even the good to do wrong."

So forgive the person who borrowed your favorite book and never returned it, forgive the person who stole the girl you liked or the guy you liked, forgive the person in your life who you can't stand being around the most. But hold righteous, indignant anger against the sins of man.

Feel righteous and justified anger at the murder of babies by abortion. Feel righteous and justified anger at the non-stop lies coming from Hollywood and the mainstream media. Feel righteous and justified anger at the corruption of so many who hold political office. Feel righteous and justified anger at unjust wars, both military and economic. Feel righteous and justified anger at the actions of those who seek to destroy the family, those who seek to destroy the country by rioting, looting, and burning down cities, and those who seek to topple Christianity. All of that is good, righteous anger. You get the idea.

Now what if you're feeling anger right now, not at the injustices I detailed above, but because of my words? What if you support the murder of babies by abortion, lies by Hollywood and the mainstream media, corrupt politicians, military and economic wars, rioting, looting, burning down cities, and the destruction of Christianity?

If that's the case, I want you to hold on to your anger for a moment. Ask yourself, who you are most angry at in your life. You might get only a vague, general feeling, but keep thinking and asking yourself and see if you can personalize it. Most likely an individual will come to mind.

It could be your father.

It could be your mother.

It could be your current or ex-boyfriend or girlfriend.

It could be God.

It could be you.

Whoever it is, feel anger toward that person, and on a scale of 1 to 10, with 10 being highest, build your anger toward that person up to a level 6.

Hold it there for a minute or so and then build your anger toward that person up to a level 8. Hold your anger toward that person at level 8 for a minute or two, and then push it all the way up to level 10.

Feel intense, level-10 anger towards that person and hold it. In a couple of minutes your anger will start to subside. You'll feel a gradual softening; a slight slipping away, and then your anger will be gone. At that point, take a few deep breaths and think about the person you felt such anger toward. With that person in mind, think about forgiving them.

I know it's hard. I know it's painful. But do it anyway. Take baby steps if you have to, but don't give up. Try to feel real forgiveness for that person. Take a full five minutes or longer here. This is an extremely important step in not only clearing your acne, but also for your overall health and appearance.

I've known people who had ugly red acne bumps all over their face for weeks and weeks try the exercise above. Within two days, their skin was completely clear. When you work on releasing anger and practicing forgiveness, amazing things happen.

A Final Word on Forgiveness

We've spoken quite a bit about the need for forgiveness. If it's a new topic for you, give it some serious thought. Most of us have more than one person we need to forgive, so the sooner we start, the better. With all the forgiveness you're now practicing don't forget to forgive the most important person of all: yourself.

It's easy to put ourselves down. When you grow up and are constantly told, "You're stupid", "you're ugly", "you'll never amount to anything", and other cheery things, it's easy to self-criticize and self-hate.

How many times have you told yourself, "How could I be so stupid?" How many times have you lowered your head and mentally kicked yourself for something you said or did? If you're like me, you've done it thousands of times.

It's easy for a person filled with self-criticism and low self-worth to manifest skin conditions, like rashes and acne. If that sounds like you, practice self-forgiveness. Be easy and gentle on yourself. Tell yourself you did the best you could with the information you had at the time.

If you hurt somebody else, apologize to that person. If you stole something from somebody, make restitution and give it back. If the person is dead, make restitution to their closest surviving relative. You don't have to explain all the details, just tell the relative that you owed the deceased person money and would like to pay it back. If you stole something from a store or business, mail it back. You can do that anonymously.

Your guilt over a person you harmed in the past just might be what's causing your acne, so it's important for you to clear that out.

In the meantime, look in the mirror and say, "I love you."

Do that literally. Say to yourself, "I love you", and "I love and approve of myself." Do those 100 times a day, if you have to, until you feel you've completely forgiven yourself.

Finally, don't forget to ask God to forgive you.

Which brings us to the next and most important chapter of this book.

Chapter Seven – Saving Your Soul - Your Ultimate Challenge

It's taken me awhile, but I've finally come to realize that most, if not all, of the illness we experience in our lives is sent to us from God.

It's sent to get our attention; to make us sit up and take notice.

Why would God do that?

Perhaps because we're not living our lives the way He wants us to. So God sends us an illness as a wakeup call.

Acne is no different.

Consider your own case. Are you truly living your life the way God wants you to?

Really?

Are you participating in any kind of behavior that would make God frown and shake His head? Are you participating in any kind of behavior that you would be embarrassed of or ashamed to admit to in His presence?

Maybe that's why you have acne.

Here's an important question: What would your life be like without acne?

Is there a certain girl you would ask out, or a certain guy you would be more open to socializing with if you didn't have acne? If so, what do you think would happen next?

Perhaps you were given acne, because without it something sinful would have occurred. Without acne, you might have dated a certain someone, engaged in mortal sin, and made her pregnant. Without acne, you might have dated a certain someone, engaged in mortal sin, and become the one pregnant.

Even worse, you might have committed the mortal sin of murder by having an abortion. Without acne, you might be engaging in mortal sin right now.

Think about those things.

Does it make more sense now why God may have sent you a case of acne in order to get your attention?

What you think is horrible now – your acne – might turn out to be the very thing that keeps you from committing mortal sin and going to hell when you die.

I told you at the very beginning that this book is different.

But I'm a Nice Person!

When I first considered the concept of God sending us wake-up calls, I thought, "That can't be me. After all, I'm spiritually perfect. And I'm a nice person."

It took me a long time to realize that I wasn't spiritually perfect, and that being a nice person doesn't count for much in Heaven.

Millions of "nice people" commit sins of lust every day.

Millions of "nice people" commit sins of omission every day by tolerating other people's sins of lust.

Millions of "nice people" are complicit in one of the worst sins of all – murder – by voting for pro-abortion politicians.

These are all very nice and kind people. They say "please" and "thank you," they welcome you into their homes and serve you tea and coffee, they smile sweetly and ask how you are doing. And yet, they are all horrible sinners.

When you really think about it, being a nice person has to be pretty low in God's pecking order. After all, it seems like people who label themselves nice are the ones committing the majority of sins and causing the most harm in the world today.

Thinking logically, a not-so-nice person (gruff, unsmiling, maybe even impolite) who loves God and honors Him by obeying the Ten Commandments is far more likely to go to Heaven than a nice person who breaks even just one Commandment.

In Hollywood, where I lived and worked for several years, I met and socialized with literally hundreds of "nice people," many of them celebrities and household names. Movie stars, television stars, television talk-show hosts, radio hosts, you name it; all of them super nice, all of them super friendly, and all of them notorious sinners on their way to hell.

Analyzing my own life, I thought back to every illness, every ache and pain I've ever experienced, including acne when I was 14-years-old, and I realized that, yes, every one of these illnesses was a wake-up call from God.

In every case, there was something going on with me that wasn't in alignment with God's wishes. In every case, the illness was sent to me either as a wake-up call to stop committing a particular sin, or as a preemptive strike to prevent me from committing a future sin.

And here's the kicker: throughout all those times, I considered myself a nice person.

How about you?

What's going on in your life that may have brought about your acne?

Take some time to think about this. If a thought or idea popped into your head while you were reading these words, write it down.

If nothing comes to mind, take a stroll in the sunshine. Think about your life; think about where you've been and where you are going. I'm willing to bet money that the reason why you developed acne will become crystal clear.

Your Life's Purpose

What is your purpose?

Why are you here?

Do you ever think about those things?

Most people believe the purpose of life is to follow your dreams. They believe that, because it's what they've been told. Nothing could be further from the truth.

The purpose of life isn't to "follow your dreams." Anyone who tells you that is an idiot. The purpose of life is to use our time here on earth to honor God and to prepare our soul to enter Heaven.

If you died today, do you think you would go to Heaven?

Really?

The sad truth – according to all available evidence - is very few people make it to Heaven. The vast majority of human beings end up burning in the fires of hell for all eternity. Think about that for a moment. Now does it make sense why God might send you a case of acne as a wakeup call?

If your own parents are concerned about your appearance and would prefer if you did not have acne, how do you think your Heavenly father feels? Of course, he doesn't want you to suffer, but what choice does he have?

The plain truth is most people refuse to listen to God unless and until they are facing some sort of crisis, usually a healing crisis. If that's the only way God can get a person's attention, then what do you expect Him to do? Of course, he's going to send that person some sort of crisis in order to get their attention. Wouldn't you?

Give this matter some thought. If you can put your finger on the reason why God might be sending you a case of acne in order to get your attention, then you're halfway there to clearing it up.

Just stop doing what He doesn't want you to do.

In some cases, it's easier said than done. But in every case it can be done.

When was the last time you prayed?

When was the last time you prayed and asked for spiritual guidance? If it's been a long time, or if you've never prayed for spiritual guidance, maybe this is a good time to do so.

The Absolute Best Advice I Can Give You

I've been straight with you throughout this entire book, and I'm going to be straight with you now: The absolute best advice I can give you is to embrace the true Catholic faith.

Now when I say the true Catholic faith, I mean just that: the true Catholic faith, which is the Catholic faith that existed publicly up until the 1960s, and still exists today in small pockets. What you see coming out of Rome today is not the true Catholic faith. What you see coming out of the schools and churches today that call themselves Catholic is not the true Catholic faith. They represent a counterfeit church, not the true Catholic Church.

A lot of people get confused by that. They see what's been happening for the last 60 years, with a succession of counterfeit Anti-Popes, counterfeit Cardinals and Bishops, and counterfeit priests that have not been validly ordained, and they say, "Wait a second. How can all this corruption, all this scandal, all this evil that I see coming from the Catholic Church represent the true church of Jesus Christ?"

The answer is they don't represent the true church of Jesus Christ, because they are not part of the true Catholic Church. They represent a counterfeit church. The true Catholic Church was infiltrated and subverted by Communists almost a century ago.

Have you ever seen a counterfeit twenty dollar bill? At first glance, it looks just like the real thing. However, when you take a closer look, it's clear that the bill is phony. And when you take a real close look, the fakery is so obvious that you wonder how you were ever fooled in the first place.

The same thing happens when you take a close look at the counterfeit church that's pretending to be Catholic. The fakery becomes so obvious that you wonder how anyone could be so easily duped.

In order to see the truth, however, it's necessary to leave emotions out of the equation and apply facts, logic, and evidence. Most people are not able or willing to do that.

You may not know this, but most people – well over 90% of the population - make their decisions about life and justify their actions based on emotions, not on facts and evidence. You might think I'm exaggerating just slightly. Trust me, I'm not. If anything, the actual figure is probably higher than 90% of the population.

When it comes to the subject at hand – the Communist subversion and takeover of the Catholic Church and the creation of a counterfeit church - the deception is so huge, so monstrous, and so evil that hundreds of millions of people simply refuse to acknowledge it.

These folks are so frightened of the truth that the majority of them refuse to even look at the evidence. In fact, just mentioning this subject causes their hands to shake and the spittle to fly from their mouths. That's how frightened they are of the truth.

As Saint Thomas Aquinas said, "The greatest charity one can do to another is to lead him to the truth."

I recommend you read the book *Outside the Catholic Church There is Absolutely No Salvation* by Brother Peter Dimond. You can find it online at www.MostHolyFamilyMonastery.com

If you can't afford to buy the book, which sells for around twenty bucks, then visit the website and read all of their free information. Watch their free videos. Immerse yourself in the truth.

Now if you're really courageous; if you're the absolute bravest of the brave, the strongest of the strong; afraid of no man and willing to do whatever it takes to achieve eternal glory, then read the book *Preparation for Death* by Saint Alphonsus Liguori.

I must warn you, it's not for the squeamish. You'll need the strength of Sampson to even begin reading it, and most people are too cowardly and too weak to do that. It's that same cowardice and that same weakness that prevents the vast majority of men and women from resisting sin and leads to their being condemned to an eternity burning in the fires of hell. All because they are too afraid to read a book or visit a website.

What about you?

Where do you stand?

You want beautiful, clear skin? You got it. Just follow the recommendations in this book.

You want to go to Heaven? You got that too. Just follow the true Catholic faith.

As always, you can email me with any questions you have.

THE END ... of this book – and the beginning of a new life ... for you.

Thank You!

THANK YOU VERY MUCH for buying this book! If you enjoyed it, please share your thoughts by posting a review where you purchased the book. People often make their book-reading decisions based on other people's reviews (I know I do), and your review of this book could be the deciding factor for someone who is wondering whether or not to read it. Even a short, one sentence review will help.

If you didn't like the book, please email me and let me know why. Perhaps I can improve it. In either case, thank you again.

If you have any questions about anything you read here, please let me know. And please let me know how fast your acne clears up. It *will* clear up if you follow the information in this book.

Mike Mains writes mystery and adventure books for sleuths of all ages. He can be reached at mainsmike@yahoo.com

The North Hollywood Detective Club Series

THE CASE OF THE HOLLYWOOD ART HEIST

Jeffrey Jones is a kid with a problem. A *lot* of problems. He's laughed at in school. The neighborhood bully has it out for him. And his parents treat him like a six-year-old. However, Jeffrey does have one ace up his sleeve: He's a master investigator.

When the brother of a classmate is arrested for stealing a valuable painting, Jeffrey and his best friend, Pablo Reyes, form The North Hollywood Detective Club and set out to rescue him from jail. Their investigation leads them to a mysterious tattoo parlor, a glamorous television star, and a 20-year-old unsolved murder.

THE CASE OF THE DEAD MAN'S TREASURE

Hired by their teacher to find the driver responsible for a hit-and-run car accident, teen detectives Jeffrey Jones and Pablo Reyes stumble upon a search for an ancient treasure. Working feverishly to decipher the clues to the treasure's location, they find themselves in a race against time with a ruthless treasure hunter who will stop at nothing to get his hands on the prize.

THE CASE OF THE CHRISTMAS COUNTERFEITERS

Two teenage detectives. One criminal mastermind. And two billion dollars in counterfeit currency. What could possibly go wrong?

While the rest of the world prepares to celebrate Christmas, Jeffrey and Pablo stumble upon a plot to flood Los Angeles with billions of dollars in counterfeit money. Together with their friends Marisol and Susie, they uncover a master criminal, his hoodlum son, and a mysterious 15-year-old girl who holds the key to the entire puzzle.

THE CASE OF THE DEADLY DOUBLE-CROSS

All Jeffrey wanted to do was help a girl at his school find her missing father. He had no way of knowing it would lead to him and his best friend being framed for murder.

Now on the run after a daring escape, and with the police closing in, Jeffrey and Pablo must solve the murder and find the real killer before the police find them.

Other Books by Mike Mains

MONKEY JOKES – A JOKE BOOK FOR KIDS!

Tickle your funny bone with these laugh-a-minute jokes for kids. Apes, cheetahs, gorillas, they're all here, ready to entertain you in the world's first and funniest collection of monkey jokes.

Are you ready for a gorillian laughs? Then stop monkeying around and get this book today!

BODYBUILDING FOR BOYS & YOUNG MEN

If you want muscles and you want them fast, this is the book for you. It's all here: what exercises to do, how often to exercise, what to eat, even how to think. A fast, fun and effective way to build your body. The bodybuilding program contained in this book has been tested hundreds of times and has a 100% success rate.

www.ingramcontent.com/pod-product-compliance
Lightning Source LLC
Chambersburg PA
CBHW070802050426
42452CB00012B/2451